Table of Contents

PREVIEW

Alkalosis is a condition concerning the pH of your blood and fluids. It occurs when your blood pH levels are imbalanced. When your blood is too acidic, it's called acidosis. When it's too alkaline, it's alkalosis.

Your blood pH should always be balanced. An increase in alkali (alkaline chemicals) is typically caused by an increase in bicarbonate, a drop in acid levels, or a decrease in carbon dioxide. The cause of the alkalosis determines what type it is.

ALKALINE DIET RECIPES

1. Sweet Potato Gnocchi

Prep Time: 15 Minutes

Cook Time: 40 Minutes

Servings: 4

Ingredients

- 2 Sweet potatos, medium 300g
- Plain flour 250g
- Egg 1
- For The Sauce:
- Plum tomatoes, fresh 500g
- Rosemary 1 tbsp/12.7g
- Rapeseed oil 1 tbsp/11g
- Salt 1 tsp/5g
- Pepper 1 tsp/2g
- Garlic powder 1 tsp/5g
- Chilli powder 1 tsp/3g
- Paprika 1 tsp/3g

Instructions

1. Start by peeling the sweet potatoes and cutting them into thirds. Place them in a saucepan, cover with water and add a pinch of salt. Boil until completely soft.

2. Drain the potatoes and mash until smooth. Leave this to cool.
3. Crack the egg into the cooled mash and mix. Add the flour bit by bit until it forms a potato-like dough. Form the dough into a rough ball and wrap in clingfilm. Leave to chill in the fridge until just before cooking.
4. While the dough cools, preheat the oven to 200°C (180°C fan.) Throw the tomatoes on to a baking dish and drizzle with the rapeseed oil and rosemary. Roast in the oven for 20-25 minutes.
5. Once the tomatoes are done, place them into a blender with all of the other herbs and spices. Blend until smooth and set aside.
6. In order to make the gnocchi, make sure that your dough is completely chilled. Remove from the fridge and place on to a floured surface to avoid sticking. For easier management divide the dough into quarters and work with one at a time. Roll out the quarter into a long, relatively thin sausage shape. Cut along the line in half inches to form little pillows of the dough. Repeat this until all the dough has been used.
7. Boil some salted water in a pan. Once bubbling, drop in the gnocchi pillows. They won't take long to cook - once they have risen to the top of the water, remove them.
8. In a separate frying pan pour in the sauce and heat until simmering. Once all the gnocchi have been boiled, tip them into the sauce and stir until everything is covered.
9. Serve hot straight from the pan. Enjoy!

Prep Time: 20 Minutes

Cook Time: 1 hrs 10 Minutes

Servings: 6

Ingredients

- Cornmeal 400g
- Semi-skimmed milk 300ml
- Eggs 2 average
- Rapeseed Oil 100ml
- Beef sizzling steak 350g
- Onion 1 Medium
- Ground black pepper 5g
- Baking powder 1 tsp

Instructions

1. Preheat the oven to 200°C for a conventional oven, 180°C for a fan oven.
2. Beat the eggs together with the milk and rapeseed oil. Add the cornmeal and mix until thoroughly combined.
3. Pour the cornbread mixture into a greased loaf tin. Bake for 40 minutes or until a skewer comes out clean when inserted into the bread.
4. Trim and discard any fat from the beef steak. Slice the steak into long, thin strips.
5. Heat up a good non-stick frying pan over a medium heat. Add the steak and fry until cooked through and

well seared. Spoon the cooked steak on to a plate and set aside.

6. Finely slice the onion. Fry the onion in the same pan you used for the steak, coating the onion in the juices left over from the meat, until the onion is soft and deeply browned.
7. Take the pan off the heat, tip the steak back into the pan with the onions and mix together.
8. Slice the cornbread as you would a loaf of bread and fill the slices with the steak and onion filling. You can make several sandwiches at the same time for the whole household, or if you'd rather have the sandwiches over several days, the cornbread and filling will stay fresh in the fridge for a few days.

Prep Time: 20 Minutes

Cook Time: 15 Minutes

Servings: 4

Ingredients

- Medium eggs, beaten 6
- Butternut squash, cubed 225g
- Feta cheese, cubed 100g
- Spinach 40g
- Cherry tomatoes 10
- Red chilli, deseeded and finely sliced 1
- Garlic clove, crushed 1
- Balsamic vinegar 1 tbsp
- Dried chilli flakes 1 tsp
- Mixed salad leaves to serve 60g

Instructions

1. Place a large non-stick pan over a medium heat and preheat the grill to 160°C.
2. Chop the butternut squash into chunks and place in a microwaveable dish for 4-5 minutes or until slightly softened.
3. Meanwhile, mix together the crushed garlic, chilli, chilli flakes and balsamic vinegar in a jug. Once mixed, pour into the pan and add the butternut squash to continue softening.
4. Add the spinach and heat until it begins to wilt.

5. Pour the eggs over the vegetable mixture and cook. When the omelette begins to cook and firm up, but still has a little raw egg on top, sprinkle over the feta chunks.
6. Remove from the heat and place under the grill for two minutes until the egg has fully set.
7. Once cooked, remove from the pan and divide into portions.
8. Serve and enjoy

Prep Time: 20 Minutes

Cook Time: 45 Minutes

Servings: 12

Ingredients

- Banana, very ripe 100g
- Skimmed milk 200ml
- Sunflower oil 30ml
- Free-range eggs, large 100g
- Orange, zest 3g
- Orange, juice 45ml
- Self-raising flour 250g
- Bicarbonate of soda 5g
- Granulated sweetener 25g
- Soft light brown sugar 30g
- Ginger, ground 2g
- Vanilla extract 2g
- Dried apricots 50g
- Dried cranberries 30g
- Desiccated coconut 10g
- Rolled oats 10g

Instructions

1. Preheat the oven 200°C/180°C Fan/Gas 4. Line a 12-hole muffin tray with large muffin cases.

2. In a bowl, mash the banana with a fork. Add the milk, sunflower oil, beaten eggs, orange zest and juice to the bowl. Mix well.
3. In a separate large bowl, mix together the flour, bicarbonate of soda, brown sugar, sweetener, ground ginger, vanilla essence and dried fruit. Add the banana mixture and mix until just combined.
4. Spoon the mixture into the muffin cases and sprinkle the desiccated coconut and rolled oats on top. Bake on the middle shelf of the oven for 15 minutes, until the muffins are golden on top and firm to the touch.
5. Remove the tray from the oven and allow the muffins to cool on a wire rack (or enjoy whilst still slightly warm).

Prep Time: 10 Minutes

Cook Time: 30 Minutes

Servings: 2

Ingredients

- Polenta (or fine cornmeal) 80g
- Boiled water 400ml
- 1 vegetable stock cube
- Hulled linseeds 80g
- Fresh spinach leaves 100g
- 3 small heritage carrots (orange, yellow, purple)
- Extra-virgin olive oil 1 tbsp
- Ground black pepper

Instructions

1. To make the croquettes: pre-heat the grill to 200°C. Dissolve the vegetable stock cube in the boiled water and place in a saucepan with the fine polenta. Bring to a gentle boil and cook for 5 minutes until the polenta mixture has a consistency similar to mashed potato.
2. Spread the polenta mixture on to a baking tray or plate to a thickness of about 1cm. Leave to cool for around 5 minutes until the mixture is cool enough to handle.

3. Place the linseeds in a small bowl. Using your hands,
    roll the cooled polenta into balls, about 1 inch in
    diameter, and roll the polenta balls in the linseeds to
    coat them.
4. Grill the croquettes for 8 minutes, shaking once, to
    lightly toast the linseed coating. Set aside.
5. Grate the heritage carrots and toss with the spinach
    leaves, olive oil and black pepper.
6. Top the salad leaves with the croquettes and sprinkle
    over any remaining linseeds to garnish. Serve and
    enjoy.

Prep Time: 10 Minutes

Cook Time: 25 Minutes

Servings: 12

Ingredients

- 8 eggs 400g
- Kale, chopped 100g
- Ricotta 125g
- Lean cooked ham, chopped 130g
- Olive oil 8g
- Onion, finely chopped 80g
- 1 garlic clove, crushed 4g
- Carrots, grated 175g
- Fresh basil, chopped 10g

Instructions

1. Heat the oven to 180°C/160°C Fan/Gas 4 and line a 12-hole muffin tin with non-stick baking paper squares.
2. Heat the oil in a non-stick frying pan set over a medium heat. Gently fry the onion for 2-3 minutes until softened. Add the garlic and grated carrot and cook, stirring, for 2 minutes or until the carrots start to soften. Add the kale and cook, stirring, until just wilted. Season with ground black pepper and set aside.

3. In a large bowl, whisk the eggs and ricotta together. Add the basil, kale mixture and ham; stir well. Spoon the mixture into the prepared muffin tin.
4. Bake for 20-25 minutes until golden, puffed and set. Set aside to cool for 5 minutes; then remove from the tin and cool on a wire rack. Serve warm or cold. Can be kept in an airtight container in the fridge for 3 days.

Prep Time: 30 Minutes

Cook Time: 55 Minutes

Servings: 4

Ingredients

- 8 skinless chicken thigh fillets 650g
- Carrots 140g
- Butternut squash 225g
- Onion, white or red 200g
- Tomatoes 250g
- Bell pepper, any colour 200g
- Rapeseed oil 1 tbsp
- Paprika 1 tbsp
- Cumin ½ tbsp
- Chilli flakes ½ tbsp
- Rosemary ½ tbsp
- Salt and pepper 1 tsp each

Instructions

1. Preheat the oven to 200°C (180°C fan).
2. First, wash all of the vegetables. Then roughly chop the carrots. Peel and de-seed the butternut squash and cut into inch chunks. Do the same with the peppers. Peel the onions and quarter along with the tomatoes.
3. Put the chopped vegetables into a large roasting dish, spreading them out evenly.

4. Lay out the chicken thighs on top of the bed of vegetables.
5. Drizzle the oil evenly over the ingredients before sprinkling on the herbs and spices. Using your hands, toss the ingredients around in the dish to make sure everything is covered.
6. Roast in the oven for 35-40 minutes.
7. Cut into the chicken thighs to make sure they are cooked properly - the juices should run clear.
8. Serve hot straight from the oven. Can be paired with a fresh salad or a small portion of wholegrain rice.

Prep Time: 30 Minutes

Cook Time: 55 Minutes

Servings: 6

Ingredients

- 1 1/2 cups Fiber One Bran Cereal
- 1/2 cup 2% milk
- 1/4 cup low-fat buttermilk
- 1 large egg yolk
- 1 Tbsp unsalted butter
- 1/2 cup unsweetened applesauce
- 1/2 cup Splenda or stevia
- 2/3 cup all purpose flour
- 2/3 cup whole wheat flour
- 1 tsp baking powder
- 1/4 tsp baking soda
- 1/4 tsp salt
- 1/2 tsp ground nutmeg
- 3 large egg whites
- 1 cup seedless raisins

Instructions

1. Place the bran cereal, milk and buttermilk in a mixing bowl. Let the mixture stand for about 20 minutes until the bran is softened. Using a whisk mash the bran until it is well blended into the milk and forms a paste. There will be some larger pieces. This is OK.

2. Preheat oven to 375°F.
3. Cream together the egg yolk and butter until smooth. Add the applesauce and the Z-Sweet or Splenda and whisk until smooth.
4. Sift the all-purpose flour, whole wheat flour, baking powder, baking soda, salt and nutmeg into the mixing bowl.
5. Sprinkle the raisins over the top of the flour mixture and then fold the flour and raisin mixture together with the bran mixture.
6. Whisk the egg whites until white and frothy (they should about triple in volume). Fold the egg whites into the muffin mixture until they are just blended in.
7. Line a standard size muffin tin with 6 muffin papers and fill each muffin paper with an equal amount of batter. Bake for 20 - 25 minutes.

Prep Time: 10 Minutes

Cook Time: 30 Minutes

Servings: 2

Ingredients

- French Toast
- 1 large egg
- 2 tsp. Grand Marnier orange liqueur
- 1/2 tsp. sugar
- 1 Tbsp. 2% milk
- 1/4 tsp. pure vanilla extract
- 1/4 cup orange juice
- 1/4 tsp. orange zest
- 4 slices sourdough bread
- 2 tsp. (per serving) unsalted butter
- Orange Honey
- 2 Tbsp. honey
- 1/2 tsp. Grand Marnier orange liqueur

Instructions

1. Place the egg, Grand Marnier, sugar, milk, vanilla extract, orange juice, and orange peel in a medium mixing bowl.
2. Whisk until well blended.
3. Heat a non-stick griddle over medium-high heat.
4. When the griddle is hot enough that a few drops of water will dance on the surface, reduce the heat to medium and place 4 slices of bread into the batter.

5. Gently dunk and turn the bread until it is well coated and slightly soaked.
6. Place the 4 slices of soaked bread on the griddle and cook for about 3 – 4 minutes. Turn and cook on the other side.
7. Cook, turning occasionally, until both sides are golden brown.
8. Depending on your stove or griddle you may need to reduce the heat slightly.
9. Remove and top with the butter and orange honey.

Prep Time: 15 Minutes

Cook Time: 35 Minutes

Servings: 2

Ingredients

- 6 Tbsp. all purpose flour
- 6 Tbsp. whole wheat flour
- 1 tsp. sugar
- 1 tsp baking powder
- 2/3 cup non-fat buttermilk
- 2 large eggs
- 1 tsp pure vanilla extract
- 2 tsp. (per serving) unsalted butter
- 1 Tbsp. (per serving) pure maple syrup

Instructions

1. Sift the all purpose flour, whole wheat flour, sugar and baking powder into a large mixing bowl.
2. Add buttermilk, eggs and vanilla extract and blend using a large whisk until smooth.
3. Heat a non-stick griddle over medium-high heat.
4. Let the batter stand for at least 2 minutes while the griddle is heating.
5. Stir once and wait another minute before placing batter on the griddle.
6. When the griddle is hot enough that a few drops of water will dance on the surface, reduce the heat to

medium and place about 1/4 cup of batter for each pancake on the griddle.

7. Allow to cook for another 1 - 2 minutes until bubbles form on the surface and burst.
8. Turn pancake and cook for about 1/2 the time of the first side until the are golden brown.
9. Remove and top with butter and maple syrup.

LUNCH

Prep Time: 10 Minutes

Cook Time: 35 Minutes

Servings: 2

Ingredients

- 1/2 tsp olive oil
- 1/4 poblano chili (seeded and diced)
- 1 ear corn (shave kernels from the cob)
- 2 green onions (sliced crosswise)
- 1/2 medium red bell pepper (seeded and julienned)
- 1/4 tsp ground cumin
- 1 tsp chili powder
- 1/8 tsp salt
- fresh ground black pepper to taste
- 1/2 cup water
- 2 Tbsp fresh cilantro leaves (chopped)
- spray oil
- 4 corn tortillas
- 2 ounces Monterey jack cheese (shredded)

Instructions

1. Heat the olive oil in a large skillet over medium heat and add the poblano. Cook for about 3 minutes until slightly soft.
2. Add the corn and increase the heat to medium-high. Cook the corn kernels, tossing frequently, until they begin to brown.
3. Add the green onions and red pepper and cook for about 3 minutes.
4. Add the cumin, chili powder, salt, pepper and cook for 2 minutes stirring continuously.
5. Add the water and cook for about 7 to 10 minutes. Stir occasionally.
6. When the water is evaporated, turn off the heat and add the cilantro. Toss until blended into the vegetable mixture.
7. Preheat a non-stick griddle or pan over medium-high heat.
8. After it is hot, spray lightly with oil and place 2 corn tortillas in the pan.
9. Top each tortilla with the 1/4 of the cheese and then 1/2 of the corn mixture. Top the corn mixture with the remaining cheese.
10. Place another tortilla on top of the corn and cheese, forming the quesadilla. Spray very lightly with oil.
11. Cook for about 5 minutes on each side, pressing down to allow the cheese to melt into the corn, holding the quesadilla together. Turn at least once.

Prep Time: 10 Minutes

Cook Time: 30 Minutes

Servings: 2

Ingredients

- 2 Tbsp. all-purpose flour or garbanzo flour
- 1/4 tsp. ground black pepper
- 2 tsp. extra virgin olive oil
- 1 tsp. unsalted butter
- 8 ounces boneless, skinless chicken breast
- 1/4 cup no salt added chicken or vegetable stock
- 2 Tbsp. white wine
- 4 tsp. capers
- 1/2 lemon (juiced)
- 1/2 tsp. lemon zest
- 1/8 tsp. salt
- 1/4 tsp. sugar

Instructions

1. Preheat the oven to 200°F.

2. Using a very sharp knife, carefully slice chicken breast on the bias into 1/2 inch thick slices (meat cut this way is called scaloppini).

3. Place the scaloppini between two sheets of plastic wrap and pound until they are about 1/4 inch thick.

4. Place the flour and pepper on a plate.

5. Place the chicken scaloppini in the flour and coat well.

6. Put the olive oil and butter in a large skillet over medium high heat and add the garlic.

7. Cook for about 2 minutes, and as the garlic begins to turn brown, add the chicken and cook for about 4 minutes on each side until browned on both sides.

8. Remove the chicken to a plate and place in the warm oven.

9. Add the chicken stock, white wine, lemon juice, lemon zest, capers, salt, and sugar to the pan and cook over medium heat, scraping the bottom of the pan until it is clean.

10. Cook for about 3 to 5 minutes until the flavor of alcohol has disappeared.

11. Add the chicken back into the pan for about 4 minutes, turning frequently.

12. The sauce will thicken to a glaze.

13. Place the chicken on a plate and top with the sauce.

Prep Time: 10 Minutes

Cook Time: 30 Minutes

Servings: 2

Ingredients

- 2 tsp. smoked paprika
- 1/8 tsp. salt
- 1/4 tsp. onion powder
- 1/4 tsp. garlic powder
- 1/4 tsp. cayenne pepper
- 1/4 tsp. fresh ground black pepper
- 1/4 tsp. dried thyme leaves
- 1/4 tsp. dried oregano leaves
- 2 4-ounce filets fresh red snapper
- 2 tsp. olive oil

Instructions

1. Place a skillet in the oven and preheat to 400°F.

2. Combine the paprika, salt, onion powder, garlic powder, cayenne pepper, black pepper, thyme, and oregano in a medium sized bowl.

3. Mix together until well blended.

4. Place the filets in the bowl and turn gently to coat the fish well with the spice mixture.

5. When the pan is hot, add the olive oil and swirl to coat the pan.

6. Place the fish in the hot pan skin side up and return the pan to the oven.

7. Cook for about 5 minutes and turn.

8. Cook for another 4 to 5 minutes and serve.

Prep Time: 20 Minutes

Cook Time: 15 Minutes

Servings: 2

Ingredients

- 1/2 tsp unsalted butter
- 1/6 green bell pepper (julienne strips)
- 2 large egg whites
- 1 large egg yolks
- 1/16 tsp salt
- 1 1/2 Tbsp water
- 3 large fresh basil leaves
- fresh ground black pepper (to taste)
- 1/4 ounce Parmigiano-Reggiano (grated)

Instructions

1. Melt the butter in a small non-stick skillet pan over medium heat. Add the peppers and cook until they are browned but not limp. Remove and set aside.
2. In a small mixing bowl whisk together the egg whites, eggs yolks, salt and water. Add ground pepper to taste.
3. Heat a medium sized non-stick skillet over medium-high heat and place the basil in the bottom and pour

the egg mixture over the top. Reduce the heat to medium heat and cook slowly. Gently slide a spatula under the eggs and carefully fold back the cooked portion so as to expose more uncooked egg to the bottom of the pan.

4. When the eggs are nearly set, add the peppers to the center (in a straight line so as to make folding easier). Fold the omelet in half over the peppers. Cook about 2 more minutes and remove.

5. Sprinkle the Parmigiano-Reggiano over the top of the omelet and then divide into two portions.

Prep Time: 10 Minutes

Cook Time: 15 Minutes

Servings: 4

Ingredients

- 3-4 tablespoons high heat oil, like grapeseed or avocado
- 2 large eggs Optional - Leave out for vegan
- 2 garlic cloves, minced
- ¾ cup green onion, chopped
- ¾ cup mixed chopped vegetables - I used 1 fresh corn on the cob and ½ red bell pepper
- 3 cups Cruciferous Crunch mix (kale/cabbage mix) or 1 bunch of kale, roughly chopped
- 2 cups chilled brown rice
- 2 tablespoons coconut aminos
- 2 teaspoons toasted sesame oil
- 2 teaspoons sweet chili sauce
- 1 teaspoon kosher salt + more to taste
- Optional: Sriracha to taste

Instructions

1. In a wok or a large cast iron skillet, heat 1-2 tablespoons (depending on the size of your pan) of oil over medium high heat. Crack 2 eggs (if using) directly into the hot pan and stir with a wooden spoon until cooked through, breaking it up into

pieces. Remove from the pan and set aside. Wipe the pan clean with a paper towel.

2. Add another 1-2 tablespoons of oil back to the pan, over medium heat. Add garlic and green onion, 1 teaspoon kosher salt, and vegetables, stirring often for 2-3 minutes.
3. Add cruciferous mixture, and cook another 2 minutes, until softened. Add chilled rice and cooked egg, mixing everything together, and spread out across the bottom of the pan, allowing it to cook without stirring for at least 30 seconds, you want the rice to get a little bit crispy. Repeat as necessary for more crispy edges. Then stir occasionally for 3 minutes over medium to medium high heat till all the rice is warmed through. Remove from heat.
4. In a small bowl or measuring cup, stir together the coconut aminos, sweet chili sauce, and toasted sesame oil. Pour the mixture into the rice, allow it to bubble, and stir till combined. Serve warm with sriracha on the side for extra spice.

Prep Time: 10 Minutes

Cook Time: 20 Minutes

Servings: 2

Ingredients

- 8 ounces Japanese eggplant (cut into 1 inch cubes)
- spray olive oil
- 1 ounce feta cheese (crumbled)
- 1 Tbsp extra virgin olive oil
- 2 Tbsp flat leaf parsley (minced)
- 1/2 tsp dried oregano
- 3 Tbsp 2% milk
- 1 medium cucumber (peeled, seeded and sliced)
- 1/4 yellow bell pepper (seeded and julienned)
- 4 cups romaine lettuce (chopped)
- 12 black olives (not oil cured)
- 2 small whole wheat or gluten-free pita bread rounds

Instructions

1. Place a large non-stick skillet in the oven and preheat to 325°F.
2. After the oven is hot spray the pan with olive oil and add the eggplant cubes. Spray lightly with olive oil and return to the oven. Cook for about twenty minutes. Check the eggplant about every five minutes tossing to

coat with the oil. Spray lightly with more oil if needed.
   Remove and let cool.
3. Place the feta cheese, oil, parsley, oregano and milk in
   a blender and puree until smooth. Place the dressing
   in the refrigerator to chill while preparing the
   vegetables.
4. After the lettuce is chopped, divide it between two
   plates and sprinkle the olives and roasted eggplant
   over the salad. Top with the cucumbers and peppers.
   Divide the dressing equally between the two salads
   and serve.

Prep Time: 25 Minutes

Cook Time: 60 Minutes

Servings: 4

Ingredients

- 4 cups water
- 1 Tbsp white wine vinegar
- 1 lb boneless skinless chicken thighs
- 4 ribs celery (diced)
- 2 cloves garlic (finely minced)
- 4 Tbsp reduced-fat mayonnaise
- 1/4 tsp salt
- fresh ground black pepper to taste

Instructions

1. Place the water and wine in a large skillet over medium heat.
2. Bring the water to a boil and then reduce the heat until the water is at a shiver.
3. Gently add the chicken thighs and poach for about 10 - 15 minutes depending on the thickness (It's best to

use an instant thermometer and remove the thighs just as they reach 160°F.)

4. Remove from the water and let the chicken rest for 3 - 5 minutes.
5. When the chicken is cool, cut the thighs into 1/2 inch cubes. Chill in the refrigerator for about 30 minutes.
6. Remove from the fridge and add the diced celery, garlic, mayonnaise, salt and pepper.
7. Fold the salad together gently and chill for another 15 minutes before serving.

Prep Time: 15 Minutes

Cook Time: 50 Minutes

Servings: 4

Ingredients

- 1 9" frozen pie crust
- 3 large eggs
- ¾ cup whole milk
- ¼ cup heavy cream
- 3 oz chevre (soft goat cheese)
- ½ cup loosely chopped fresh spinach
- 1 shallot, chopped
- ¼-1/2 teaspoon salt and black pepper
- fresh thyme (optional)

Instructions

1. Remove pie crust from freezer and allow it to warm while you preheat your oven. When softened a bit, poke holes all around the crust with the tines of a fork. If you want your crust to not puff up even more, fill it with pie weights or beans. Pre-bake your pie crust according to package directions (mine was 425 degrees F for 15-20 minutes) on the bottom ⅓rd of your oven, until very lightly browned.
2. Meanwhile, mix together the eggs, milk, cream and whisk till combined. Then add goat cheese (crumble with your fingers), spinach, and chopped shallot with

kosher salt and black pepper and stir. The goat cheese will not fully combine, but that's ok, it will melt down.

3. Remove pre-baked pie crust from the oven, change the temperature to 400 degrees F, and pour in the filling. It's really ok if you pie bottom breaks a part a bit, you won't be able to tell once it's baked.

4. Bake at 400 degrees F for about 50 minutes, until the center is puffed up. It should have just a slight jiggle, not a wave, when you move it around. Allow it to set/cool for about 5-10 minutes before eating. I LOVE a little fresh thyme leaves on top if you have them on hand.

Prep Time: 10 Minutes

Cook Time: 20 Minutes

Servings: 4

Ingredients

- 2 pounds salmon, skin-on and bones removed
- olive oil, salt, and pepper
- Mango Salsa
- 1 large mango if buying fresh, you want it to be firm with a slight give when pressed, like an avocado.
- ¼ cup fresh cilantro
- ½ red bell pepper, chopped
- 1 small shallot, chopped
- ½ watermelon radish chopped (or regular red radish if you can't find)
- ¼ green jalapeno, seeds and membrane removed, minced the seeds and membrane contain the most heat. You can adjust accordingly to your personal heat level preference.
- 1 teaspoon distilled white vinegar
- Salt to taste

Instructions

1. Use a peeler to peel the skin from the mango. Slice around the largest diameter of your mango, avoiding the pit. Add chopped cilantro, red bell pepper, radish, vinegar, and chopped shallot. If using jalapeno, remove the seeds and membrane first, then dice into

small pieces. If you'd like a little salt, I added about ¼ tsp. You can taste it and see what you think it needs. Cover and place the salsa in the fridge. This can be made 1 day ahead.

2. Turn grill to high heat till it reaches 425-450 degrees F. Drizzle salmon with extra virgin olive oil on both sides and sprinkle with some kosher salt and pepper. Place on top of a sheet of tin foil, skin side down.

3. Once grill has reached desired temperature, place salmon with the foil directly on the heat. Close the cover to the grill and cook for 8-12 minutes or until the fat *just starts* to render on top of the salmon. If you allow it to fully render, it will be overdone.

4. If salmon has been cooked all the way through, serve immediately. If middle of filet is still raw, allow salmon to rest 5 minutes loosely covered in aluminum before serving.

Prep Time: 25 Minutes

Cook Time: 10 Minutes

Servings: 4

Ingredients

Marinated Salmon

- 1½ pounds fresh salmon, skin off, cut into 1 inch cubes
- ⅓ cup coconut aminos
- 1 tablespoon toasted sesame oil
- 1 garlic clove, minced

Bowls

- 2 tablespoons distilled white vinegar
- 1 tablespoon coconut aminos
- 8 oz bag shredded cabbage/slaw mix
- 20 oz bag microwavable rice, brown or white
- 1 cup shredded carrots
- ½ english (seedless) cucumber, sliced
- 2 tablespoons toasted sesame seeds and/or panko

Spicy Mayo

- ⅓ cup mayonnaise
- 1 tablespoon sriracha
- 1 teaspoon distilled white vinegar or lime juice

Instructions

1. In a medium bowl, combine salmon, coconut aminos, toasted sesame oil, and garlic. Stir to combine and place in the fridge for at least 30 minutes to marinate.

2. Meanwhile, stir together the mayonnaise, sriracha, and vinegar - adjusting to your taste for spice level. Set aside. Stir together the coconut aminos and vinegar, then toss the cabbage with the mixture, thoroughly coating the cabbage, and set in the refrigerator till ready to use. Microwave the rice and chop the vegetables.

3. Over medium heat, add salmon to a large non-stick or carbon steel pan, leaving space between pieces to sear. Adjusting heat to medium-medium high to sear on first side for about 2 minutes till a nice caramelization forms on the outside. Don't mess with the salmon or move it around, or it may stick and not sear properly.

4. Using tongs, flip salmon to the other side and cook another 2 minutes till cooked through to a medium temperature (or cook longer if you want it to be cooked through). You may need to work in batches, so set a plate with a paper towel next to the pan and remove the salmon pieces as they're finished.

5. Build your bowl - Add rice and slaw to the bottom, then top with carrots, cucumber, and salmon. Drizzle with spicy mayo and top with panko and/or sesame seeds.

DINNERS

Prep Time: 15 Minutes

Cook Time: 10 Minutes

Servings: 6

Ingredients

Halloumi Couscous Salad

- 1 cup couscous
- 2 fresh corn cobs, kernels removed1 cup seedless cucumber, chopped
- 2 green onion, chopped
- ½ 15oz can low sodium black beans
- ¾ cup chopped tomatoes
- 1½ cups arugula or spinach (or just a large handful)
- 8 oz halloumi cheese

Creamy Dijon Dressing

- 1 tablespoon shallot, minced
- ⅓ cup extra virgin olive oil
- 2 tablespoons vinegar
- 1 tablespoon apple juice
- 2 teaspoons dijon mustard
- 1 teaspoon mayonnaise
- 2 teaspoons honey
- Salt and black pepper to taste

Instructions

1. In a large, shallow pan with a lid, add 1 cup of water and bring to a simmer over medium heat. Stir in couscous and corn kernels, cover, and turn off the heat. Let it sit for 10 minutes, then remove lid and fluff with a spoon.
2. Meanwhile place all the ingredients for the dressing in a small mason jar and shake till creamy and well-mixed (or whisk). Add the cucumber, green onions, black beans, tomatoes, and arugula to a large bowl, along with the couscous.
3. Carefully use a paper towel soaked with vegetable or avocado oil to rub the grill grates and preheat the grill to medium high heat. Add halloumi cheese, sliced in half if very thick, and grill for 4-5 minutes per side or until grill marks form and the cheese begins to soften inside.
4. Toss couscous and vegetables with a little bit of the dressing (taste and see how much you like before adding in the entire dressing). Season with salt and freshly cracked black pepper to taste, but go easy on the salt because halloumi will fill in what you're missing. Serve with the halloumi in whole pieces or sliced.
5. Quinoa can be substituted for couscous for a gluten free option.
6. For extra flavor, I love to simmer vegetable broth instead of water which helps flavor the couscous even more.
7. Trader Joe's has the best price on halloumi that I have seen.
8. For a low sodium alternative, use mozzarella balls instead of halloumi (but don't grill them).

9. Wait to toss the dressing till the end so the vegetables
don't get soggy.
10. For migraine-friendly, use a sulfite-free dijon
mustard.

Prep Time: 5 Minutes

Cook Time: 10 Minutes

Servings: 4

Ingredients

- Honey Chipotle Chicken Breasts
- 1 ¼-1/2 pounds thin sliced boneless, skinless chicken breasts, or chicken breasts pounded to ½-3/4" thickness
- 1 teaspoon chipotle chili powder
- ½ teaspoon smoked paprika
- ½ teaspoon cumin
- ½ teaspoon garlic powder
- ½ teaspoon kosher salt
- 2 tablespoons honey
- 3 tablespoons olive oil
- Sandwich Toppings
- 4 large buns, lightly toasted if desired
- fresh cucumber, sliced into coins
- fresh red radish, sliced into coins
- Bibb or romaine lettuce leaves
- 1 shallot, thinly sliced

Spicy Mayo

- ¼ cup mayonnaise For migraine-friendly mayo,
- sriracha sauce to taste For migraine-friendly srirachas,

Instructions

1. In a large dish or ziploc bag, combine the chipotle chili powder, smoked paprika, cumin, garlic powder, and salt. Add honey and olive oil and mix till combined. Add chicken and thoroughly coat both sides in the spice mixture. Cover (if using a large dish) and place in the fridge for at least 30 minutes and up to 24 hours.
2. Prep your grill to medium heat. If using coals, place them on one side of the grill. Cook chicken off the indirect heat for about 8-10 minutes (flip over at about the 5 minute mark or until grill marks form) until the chicken is cooked through and the internal temperature registers 165 degrees F. Remove from heat and cover with tin foil to rest.
3. Prepare the sandwiches. Lightly toast the buns, if you'd like. Coat both sides with spicy mayo, slices of radish, cucumber, and shallots. Top with grilled chicken breasts and lettuce. Serve warm.
4. I prefer to use air-chilled chicken for better flavor and texture.
5. Make sure your chicken is grilled off direct heat unless you're using a grill pan. Chicken should register a temperature of 165 degrees to be cooked thoroughly.
6. If you're not following a low tyramine migraine diet, feel free to add avocado slices.
7. If gluten free or paleo, try this in lettuce wraps or on top of a salad with corn, black beans, and radish.

Prep Time: 5 Minutes

Cook Time: 15 Minutes

Servings: 4

Ingredients

- 2 pounds boneless, skinless chicken breasts or thighs
- 3 tablespoons extra virgin olive oil or avocado oil
- 3 tablespoons pomegranate juice or tart cherry juice
- 1 ½ teaspoons cumin
- ¾ teaspoon chili powder
- 1 teaspoon smoked paprika
- ½ teaspoon kosher salt
- 3 large garlic cloves, minced

Instructions

1. In a gallon sized bag, combine the oil, juice, cumin, chili powder, smoked paprika, salt, and minced garlic cloves. Smoosh around to mix everything up. Drop in the chicken breasts (see note on size of chicken breasts), and marinate for at least 2 hours, up to 12 hours.
2. Preheat the grill to medium/high heat (about 400-450 degrees F) and place a little bit of oil onto a paper towel. Using tongs, rub the towel on the grill grates to oil them, being careful to avoid excess oil flare ups. A little bit of oil goes a long way! Place chicken breasts on the grill, close the grill lid, and cook for about 5-7

minutes per side, or until grill marks form and the chicken reaches an internal temp of 165 degrees Fahrenheit. The chicken will release easily from the grill grates when it's ready to be flipped.

3. Remove from the grill and cover with foil. When ready, slice the chicken breasts and serve warm.
4. If using thin-sliced chicken breasts, which marinate and cook much faster, cook for about 4-5 minutes per side.
5. To get thin chicken breasts - run a sharp knife down the middle center of the chicken (sideways) or use a mallet to pound to about ½ inch thickness.
6. A grill pan will also work if you don't own a charcoal or gas grill. See post for instructions for baking and pan-searing chicken.
7. This marinade will keep up to a week without the chicken. Use for other types of meat like pork or flank steak, or brush onto grilled vegetables.

Prep Time: 15 Minutes

Cook Time: 35 Minutes

Servings: 4

Ingredients

- 1 pound tomatillos
- 3-4 garlic cloves
- 1 poblano, de-seeded and sliced in half
- ⅔ cup chopped shallots
- 4 cups vegetable or chicken broth
- 2 teaspoons cumin
- 2 teaspoons oregano
- 1 teaspoon coriander
- 1 teaspoon kosher salt
- ¾ pound cooked, shredded chicken I use a "naked" rotisserie chicken, meaning no spices added
- ½ cup fresh cilantro, chopped
- fresh tortillas or tortilla chips

Instructions

1. Preheat broiler to high heat. Remove paper skins and stems from tomatillos and wash under warm water to remove sticky residue. You can leave the garlic skin on for broiling. Place the tomatillos, garlic, and poblano on a baking sheet and broil about 6-10 inches away from heat for 6 minutes. Flip tomatillos and remove

the poblano and garlic if softened and charred in spots. Peel skin off garlic. Continue broiling the tomatillos until softened and charred in spots, another 6 minutes.

2. Meanwhile prep a large soup pot. Add the charred tomatillos, garlic, and poblano to the pot along with the chopped shallots and saute over medium heat about 2 minutes until the shallots have softened. Add 4 cups of broth, cumin, oregano, coriander, and salt. Stir to combine and bring to a boil, then decrease the heat to simmer for 10 minutes. Add chopped cilantro. With an immersion blender, blend the soup in the pot till it reaches your desired consistency (I like mine smooth). Stir in chicken and adjust any seasonings to your liking.

3. To serve, top with crispy tortilla chips, or toast fresh tortillas brushed on both sides with a little bit of olive oil at 400 degrees F for about 7-10 minutes until light brown. They'll crisp up as they cool.

4. Canned tomatillos can be substituted for fresh, but fresh are preferable.

5. See notes in post for gluten free/vegetarian/vegan.

6. You can find naked chickens at Sprouts, Whole Foods, and Fresh Market but any plain, cooked chicken will do.

Prep Time: 5 Minutes

Cook Time: 10 Minutes

Servings: 4

Ingredients

Blackened Cod

- 2 teaspoons chili powder
- 1 teaspoon garlic powder
- ½ teaspoon oregano
- 1 teaspoon paprika
- 1 teaspoon kosher salt (or less, if low sodium)
- ¼ teaspoon cayenne
- 1 ½ pounds fresh cod filet, skin removed
- mild oil or butter for frying

Coleslaw

- ⅓ cup mayonnaise
- 1 tablespoon distilled white vinegar
- 1 teaspoon honey
- ¼ teaspoon cumin
- 8 oz shredded cabbage mix
- 1 green onion, chopped
- ¼ cup shredded carrots
- salt and pepper to taste

Instructions

1. In a small bowl, mix together the chili powder, garlic powder, oregano, paprika, salt, and cayenne (if using). Cut cod into 4 servings of filets and pat both sides with the spice mixture.
2. Using a cast iron pan, heat 1-2 tablespoons of butter or oil over medium high heat. When oil is shimmering and hot, add the seasoned cod and sear for 5 minutes, until blackened and crispy. Flip and cook another 4-5 minutes until blackened and cooked through.
3. Meanwhile combine the mayonnaise, vinegar, honey and cumin and whisk till smooth. Toss with the cabbage, green onion, and carrots. Place in the fridge for at least 5 minutes to allow flavors to combine and cabbage to soften. Serve coleslaw under the fish.
4. If you don't like your fish spicy, simply omit the cayenne. It will still have some heat from the chili powder, but not be too spicy.
5. For low sodium, you can edit the amount of salt used.
6. If you don't own a cast iron pan, it's ok. You may just not get as great of a dark crust on the fish. However, it will be important to preheat your pan to high heat.

Prep Time: 5 Minutes

Cook Time: 20 Minutes

Servings: 3

Ingredients

- 1 pound ground beef
- Salt and black pepper
- Olive oil
- 8 oz cauliflower rice
- ½ teaspoon chili powder
- ½ teaspoon cumin
- ½ teaspoon smoked paprika
- 2 zucchini squash, cut into cubes
- 1 cup spinach
- 2 large eggs
- 2 green onion, chopped
- Salsa Verde or any salsa

Instructions

1. In a large non stick pan, cook ground beef over medium high heat, stirring frequently, till cooked through and crumbly - about 5-6 minutes total. Season with a pinch of salt and pepper, then remove from the pan and set aside.
2. In the same pan, add a teaspoon of olive oil and cauliflower rice, along with the chili powder, cumin,

and smoked paprika. Cook for 1-2 minutes over medium heat, then add the zucchini, cooking another 2-3 minutes till just barely softened. Add ¼ teaspoon of kosher salt and a pinch of fresh pepper and set aside.

3. Carefully wipe out the pan with a paper towel and add another teaspoon of olive oil over medium high heat. Crack the eggs and carefully lay them into the pan so the yolk doesn't break apart. Allow the egg to cook till the whites are set, then flip and cook another 20-40 seconds for an over easy/medium egg. Meanwhile, use the other side of pan to wilt the spinach just slightly.

4. In a bowl, add the cauliflower rice and zucchini, top with the ground beef, then add the eggs and spinach. Taste and adjust any seasonings and then add your favorite salsa and top with chopped green onions.

5. This is my favorite salsa verde, but I really like Tacodeli's Salsa Verde for a store-bought option (found at Whole Foods).

6. I used Trader Joe's fresh cauliflower rice for this recipe and used ½ a bag, approximately 8oz.

7. For extra flavor, also season your beef using this ground beef taco seasoning recipe.

8. If you're not following a migraine diet or have reintroduced foods, sliced avocado is a

9. wonderful addition, as well as a little bit of lime juice on top.

Prep Time: 15 Minutes

Cook Time: 20 Minutes

Servings: 6

Ingredients

Quinoa:

- 2 cups quinoa
- 2 cups vegetable broth
- 2 cups water

Ground Beef Stir Fry

- 1 tablespoon toasted sesame oil
- 2 pounds ground beef
- ¾ cup coconut aminos
- 3-4 garlic cloves, minced
- 10 oz broccoli florets, torn into smaller pieces
- 1 cup shredded carrots
- 4 green onions, sliced
- salt and pepper
- Optional Roasted Sweet Potato
- 2 sweet potatoes, peeled and cut into ½ inch cubes.

Instructions

1. If roasting the sweet potato, preheat oven to 425 degrees. Roast for 40 minutes, flipping halfway through, till browned on all sides.

2. Start by preparing the quinoa (or brown rice), bring quinoa and 2 cups of broth and 2 cups of water to a boil, cover and simmer for 15-20 minutes until the liquid is absorbed and it's fluffy. Season with salt and pepper to taste

3. In a large pan, add ground beef and cook over medium heat, stirring frequently until cooked through - about 5 minutes. Drain any excess fat. Add sesame oil, garlic, and coconut aminos and bring to a simmer. Stir in broccoli and carrots, mixing often. Cook until softened about 5-6 minutes. Add salt and pepper to taste.

4. Meanwhile heat a small pot over high heat until boiling. Carefully lower in eggs with a spoon and boil for 6 ½ minutes. Remove and dunk into an ice bath or under cold water. Carefully peel the egg, making sure to not puncture the yolk.

5. Spoon quinoa into a bowl and top with the ground beef, vegetables, and sauce. Cut egg in half and top with green onion. Garnish with sesame seeds, if desired.

6. This recipe makes 6 very large portions. Enough for a filling lunch or dinner.

7. I like to use 80/15 ground beef for this recipe, but choose whatever you prefer.

8. If in a hurry, skip the sweet potatoes for a quick 30 minute meal.

9. Salt balances the sweetness of the coconut aminos, so if you think it's too sweet, add more salt or some acidity, like vinegar.

Prep Time: 15 Minutes

Cook Time: 20 Minutes

Servings: 4

Ingredients

- Moroccan-Inspired Grilled Chicken
- 2 pounds boneless, skinless chicken breasts pounded to ¾ inch thickness
- ⅓ cup extra virgin olive oil
- 2 large garlic cloves minced
- 1 teaspoon honey
- 2½ teaspoon paprika
- 1½ teaspoon cumin
- ½ teaspoon coriander
- ¼ teaspoon ginger
- ¼ teaspoon cinnamon
- ¼ teaspoon turmeric
- 1 kosher salt
- ¼ teaspoon freshly ground black pepper
- Pomegranate Couscous
- 2 tablespoons olive oil
- 1 large shallot, chopped
- 1 cup vegetable or chicken broth
- 1 teaspoon paprika
- ¾ cup Moroccan-style couscous (not Israeli)
- ¼ cup roasted, unsalted sunflower seeds
- ⅓ cup pomegranate seeds
- 2 tablespoons flat leaf parsley, chopped
- ¼ teaspoon kosher salt and black pepper (each)

Instructions

1. Place all the ingredients in a large ziplock bag or shallow dish and marinate at least 30 minutes to an hour, up to 24 hours total.
2. Brush grill pan with olive oil and heat to medium-high heat. Add marinated chicken and sear on first side 4 minutes. Flip and sear on other side 3-4 minutes (mine took 3). The internal temperature should be at least 165 degrees. Wrap in tin foil until you're ready to serve. For full size chicken breasts, grill for about 7-8 minutes per side.
3. Meanwhile, in a large, deep pan (that has a lid) warm olive oil over medium high heat and sauté shallot for 1 minute. Add broth and paprika and bring to a simmer.
4. Remove the pan from the heat and add couscous. Cover with the lid and allow to sit for 10 minutes. Remove lid and fluff couscous with a fork. Add pomegranate seeds, sunflower seeds, and parsley. Season to taste.
5. The longer the chicken is marinated, the more flavorful it will be...up to a point! After 24 hours, the texture of the chicken can change so limit it to within 24 hours.
6. This chicken can also be grilled on a grill pan or simply seared on both sides till cooked through.
7. For gluten free, substitute couscous with quinoa or brown rice and cook according to package directions before mixing with the spices and seeds.

Prep Time: 15 Minutes

Cook Time: 1hrs 20 Minutes

Servings: 6

Ingredients

- 2.75 pounds boneless beef chuck roast cut into bite sized pieces
- Splash of olive oil
- 2 tablespoons butter or olive oil
- 2 large shallots, chopped
- 2 celery stalks, chopped
- 3 carrots, peeled and chopped
- 3 garlic cloves, minced
- 3 yukon gold potatoes, cut into 1" pieces
- 2 tablespoons flour
- 2 sprigs fresh rosemary
- ½ teaspoon dried thyme
- 2 bay leaves
- 5 cups low sodium beef or vegetable broth
- Salt and pepper

Instructions

1. In a large dutch oven, splash a bit of olive oil and turn to medium high heat. Season beef with kosher salt and black pepper. Add chopped beef chuck roast in batches, leaving enough space so it browns and doesn't steam. Brown on all sides, about 5-6 minutes total. Repeat with any leftover meat.

2. Remove the meat and leave the drippings. Add 2 tablespoons butter or olive oil to the dutch oven along with shallots, celery, and carrots. Stir occasionally over medium heat until softened, about 3 minutes. Add garlic and mix into the vegetables. Then add the potatoes and beef. Stir in flour with a wood spoon until fully mixed in, coating all the beef and vegetables.

3. Stir in rosemary, thyme, bay leaves, ½ teaspoon kosher salt, and finally all the broth (or any other liquid additions you're using). Bring everything to a boil over high heat and reduce heat to low. Cover and cook on low heat (or enough for a low simmer) for about 1.5 hours or until the beef is tender and flavors have combined. Taste and adjust any seasonings. Remove bay leaves and rosemary stalks before serving.

Prep Time: 20 Minutes

Cook Time: 30 Minutes

Servings: 4

Ingredients

- ¼ cup butter
- 2 large shallots, chopped
- 2 large carrots, chopped small (1 cup)
- ¼ cup all purpose flour (gluten free if needed)
- 3 cups vegetable broth
- 1 ½ cups whole milk
- 1 head broccoli chopped into florets (about 2 full cups florets)
- 5 oz Boursin Garlic & Herb cheese
- ¾ teaspoon kosher salt (or omit for lower sodium)
- ½ teaspoon black pepper

Instructions

1. In a large, heavy pot (I used a 5 ½ quart pot), melt the butter over medium heat and stir in chopped shallots and carrots. Saute for about 2 minutes until they are fragrant and more tender, stirring often. Add ¼ cup of flour and coat the vegetables. Pour in about ½ cup of broth and whisk till the flour gets incorporated and smooth. Then add the rest of the broth as well as the whole milk. Bring to a low simmer for 8-10 minutes,

allowing it to thicken. Do not start to boil, otherwise your milk might curdle (especially if using a low fat option instead).

2. Add the broccoli florets and cook for another 5 minutes until softened. Off the heat, stir in Boursin cheese until smooth and creamy. Taste and adjust any seasonings, like salt and pepper if needed.

Prep Time: 20 Minutes

Cook Time: 30 Minutes

Servings: 4

Ingredients

- 8 slices whole wheat or seed bread
- 4 slices mozzarella cheese
- ⅓ cup fresh basil leaves
- ⅓ cup mayonnaise
- 1 pound turkey breast sliced
- 1 whole roasted red pepper
- Fresh spinach leaves or lettuce

Instructions

1. Preheat broiler to low heat. Place the bread on a sheet pan and toast on one side for about 1 minute. Flip and place mozzarella cheese on the opposite side and broil again for 1 minute until melted.
2. Meanwhile in a small food processor (or just finely chop and mix), combine the basil and mayonnaise (and parsley if using) and process until almost smooth.
3. Spread pesto mayo on the other side of the bread. Top with turkey, roasted red peppers, spinach or lettuce, and freshly cracked pepper.

www.ingramcontent.com/pod-product-compliance
Lightning Source LLC
Chambersburg PA
CBHW072339270726
48659CB00022B/2043